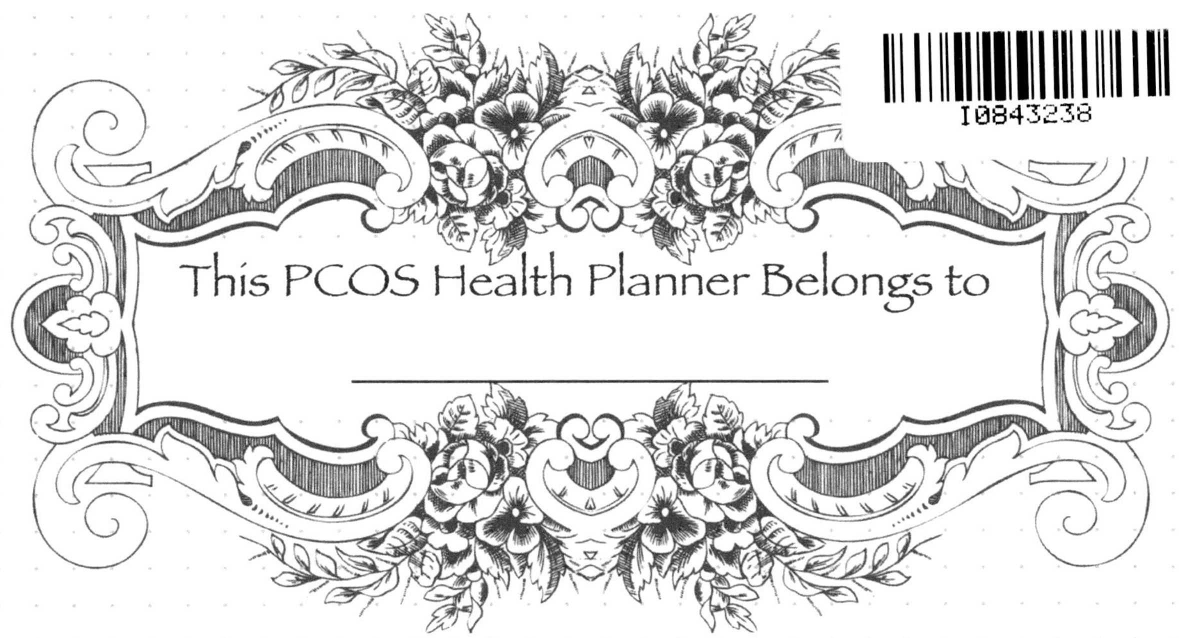
This PCOS Health Planner Belongs to

<table>
<tr><td>

New Career Goals

</td><td>

Self-Love Goals

</td></tr>
<tr><td>

Exercise Goals

</td><td>

New Activity Goals

</td></tr>
<tr><td>

Trip Planning Goals

</td><td>

Self-Care Goals

</td></tr>
</table>

January Events | February Events

April Events | March Events

May Events | June Events

<table>
<tr><td>

Summer Goals

</td><td>

Travel Goals

</td></tr>
<tr><td>

New Mindset Goals

</td><td>

Fall Activity Goals

</td></tr>
<tr><td>

Holiday Goals

</td><td>

New Year Goals

</td></tr>
</table>

<table>
<tr><td>

July Events

</td><td>

August Events

</td></tr>
</table>

<table>
<tr><td>

September Events

</td><td>

October Events

</td></tr>
</table>

<table>
<tr><td>

November Events

</td><td>

December Events

</td></tr>
</table>

- ## What exactly is PCOS ? Polycystic ovary syndrome is a commonly known hormonal disorder that effects women who are of the age of reproduction. It can start in young girls at as early of the age of 11 and effect women all the way up to the age of 50. But the most common cases occur between the age of 18-45.

- ## Although the exact cause of PCOS is not known - If you are experiencing symptoms like: severe breakouts of acne, excess body or facial hair, male pattern baldness (thinning on the top or front of your head), infrequent or irregular menstrual cycles, weight issues due to hormonal imbalances, unexplained hypertension, skin discoloration, increased feelings of anxiety or stress, bouts of depression or if PCOS runs in your family. I would recommend seeing your Doctor. Once diagnosed there are things that you can start doing on your own to help reduce the risk of experiencing any long term complications in the future.

- ## Adapt a Regular Consumption/Eating Schedule - Eating at regularly scheduled intervals will program your body to better process foods after surgery. It will also help to regulate your hormones, reduce body weight, stabilize blood sugar & cholesterol levels, & regulate sleeping patterns.

- ## Adapt a Regular Exercise Schedule - The best time to Exercise is whenever you can. But by adapting a schedule it will make it easier to adjust. For most people the best time if possible to exercise is in the mornings, because you will rarely have things that interfere with your schedule. Exercise also increases your productivity & mental clarity, releases endorphins and sparks your metabolism, helps reduce stress & promotes healthier skin. Another benefit of morning exercise is, it gets your workout done so that you can focus on other things throughout the day.

- **Genetics/Heredity -** Studies show that certain Genes may be linked to PCOS. For instance insulin resistance from either side of the family can be passed down & can be an attributing cause, and although some women don't experience symptoms until their late 20's or early 30's, studies show that if you have PCOS you were born with it.

- **Physical Changes & Problems-** For the most part the problem is that your body is producing too much androgen. This is why it is harder for you to become pregnant, and why you are growing excess hair, and if not treated PCOS can lead to more serious (if those weren't serious enough) problems like heart disease & even cancer. Another effect of PCOS are the cyst that basically attack your ovaries, these can lead to major hormonal imbalances. But wait it gets worse! PCOS also increases your risk for strokes & can possibly lead to death...

- **Complications -** There are also other complications that are associated with PCOS which include:

    - Abnormal Uterine Bleeding

    - Endometrial Cancer (Cancer of your Uterine lining)

    - Gestational Diabetes (aka Pregnancy induced ↑ BP)

    - Infertility

    - Metabolic Syndrome

    - Miscarriage or Premature Births

    - Nonalcoholic Steatohepatitis (A fatty liver disease)

    - Obesity can also complicate PCOS by exacerbating the metabolic, psychological & reproductive features of the disease.

- **Lifestyle Changes -** Although your Doctor may prescribe you medications, to regulate your menstrual cycle, help you ovulate, or reduce hair growth. Be aware that with every new thing that you put into your body, there will come more side effects & symptoms to deal with. So for the most part you need to adapt a healthy lifestyle, so that you can stimulate normal processes on your own, and be able to deal with the added stress from the medications.

- **Avoid Negative Stress -** Avoid negative people, negative self-talk and negative thinking. Negative thinking triggers hormones in our bodies that can lead to bouts of anxiety, depression & mood disorders. It's important to get in at least 30 minutes of exercise every day to help your body & mind detox & release stress through that avenue. Exercise will also help lower your blood sugar levels, help prevent insulin resistance and help you to manage your weight. I recommend meeting with a professional that can help you put together a resistance/weight program and a complimenting cardio program as well.

- **Journal -** Utilize your journal in the back to vent & release your thoughts & emotions when needed. Journaling will also help you reach your goals, strengthen your self-discipline & increase self-confidence. The last thing that you want to do, is let your emotions pile up.

- **Cookbook -** Utilize your cookbook to log meals that are healthy & that give you good energy throughout the day. Most Doctors recommend Low Carb Meals. But I would say, opt for more complex carbs & whole grains. But overall we all metabolize foods differently. So the key is to write down how you feel approximately 1 hour after eating this will give you the best feedback in regards to what you should or shouldn't be eating. If you feel like you have enough energy for another hour or two, I would say that is a good meal for you, so log in your recipe book. If not, try adding a little more healthy fats, or protein. But not both at the same time.

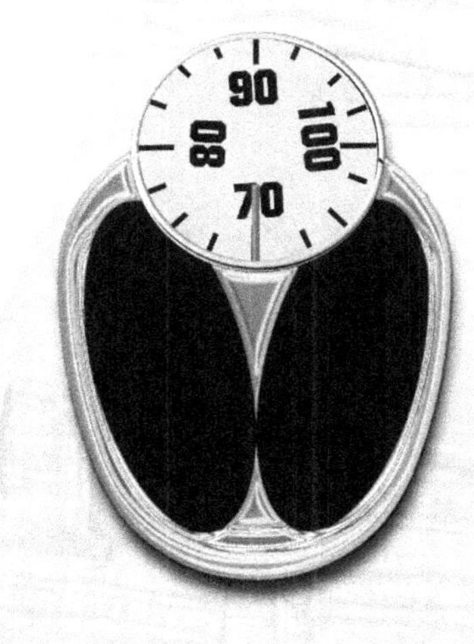

Measurements

Weight		Body Mass Index (BMI)	
Body Fat %		Water Weight	
Bust		Muscle Weight	
Chest		**Ok How are we Looking?**	
Waist			
Hips			
Thighs			
Calves			
Upper Arm			
Fore Arm			

How do you feel Overall about your measurements?

How do you feel Overall?

What do you think will be your biggest challenge?

What can you do to overcome that challenge?

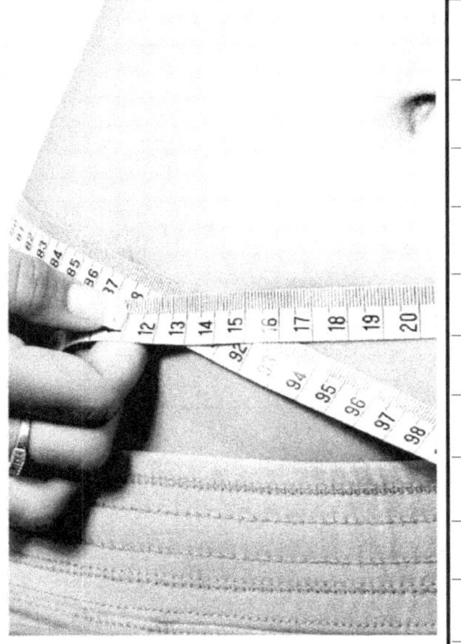

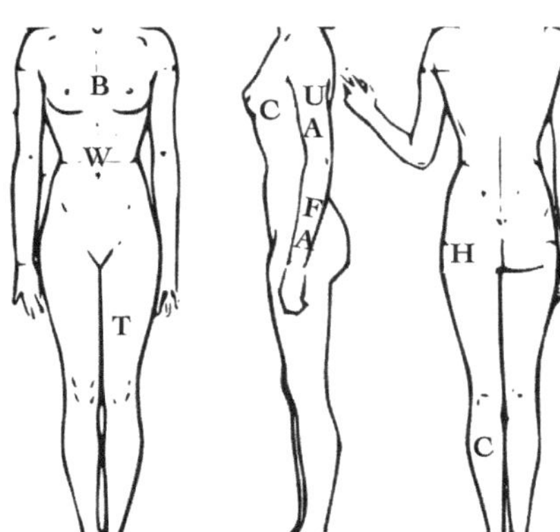

Monthly
Period Tracker

Cycle Day	January	February	March	April	May	June	July	August	September	October	November	December	Mode	Normal/Cool	Heavy/Stress
1															
2															
3															
4															
5															
6															
7															
8															
9															
10															
11															
12															
13															
14															

Cycle

Sprinkle

Light

Medium

Heavy

Notes/Comments

Vacations
Important Dates

Monthly
Ovulation Tracker

Cycle Day	January	February	March	April	May	June	July	August	September	October	November	December	Mode	Period Started/P	Ovulation/OT
1													P		
2															
3															
4															
5															
6															
7															
8															
9															
10															
11														ot	
12														ot	
13														ot	
14														ot	
15														ot	
16														ot	
17														ot	
18															
19															
20															
21															
22															
23															
24															
25															
26															
27															
28															
29															
30															
31															

30 Day Misc. Habit Tracker

Day						Smoking									
1															
2															
3															
4															
5															
6															
7															
8															
9															
10															
11															
12															
13															
14															
15															
16															
17															
18															
19															
20															
21															
22															
23															
24															
25															
26															
27															
28															
29															
30															
31															

30 Day Misc. Habit Tracker

Day

| 1 |
| 2 |
| 3 |
| 4 |
| 5 |
| 6 |
| 7 |
| 8 |
| 9 |
| 10 |
| 11 |
| 12 |
| 13 |
| 14 |
| 15 |
| 16 |
| 17 |
| 18 |
| 19 |
| 20 |
| 21 |
| 22 |
| 23 |
| 24 |
| 25 |
| 26 |
| 27 |
| 28 |
| 29 |
| 30 |
| 31 |

Snacks

30 Day Misc. Habit Tracker

Day

| 1 |
| 2 |
| 3 |
| 4 |
| 5 |
| 6 |
| 7 |
| 8 |
| 9 |
| 10 |
| 11 |
| 12 |
| 13 |
| 14 |
| 15 |
| 16 |
| 17 |
| 18 |
| 19 |
| 20 |
| 21 |
| 22 |
| 23 |
| 24 |
| 25 |
| 26 |
| 27 |
| 28 |
| 29 |
| 30 |
| 31 |

January 2020

Sun	Mon	Tue	Wed	Thu	Fri	Sat
Feelings Events Dates	Notes Appoint. Birthdays	31	1	2	3	4
5	6	7	8	9	10	11
12	13	14	15	16	17	18
19	20 MLK	21	22	23	24	25
26	27	28	29	30	31	1

Monthly Overview/Notes

____

____

____

Put a check mark if you ate on time!	Brkfast		Lunch		Dinner	
Monday						
Tuesday	✓					
Wednesday						
Thursday						
Friday						
Saturday						
Sunday						

1 hr After each meal write an emoji for how you feel as far as energy, happy for good sad for bad!

Habit Tracker

Positive Pick New	Negative Pick Old

Use The initials of each day to track Your New & Old Habits

Water Intake	64oz. 's
Monday	
Tuesday	
Wednesday	
Thursday	
Friday	
Saturday	
Sunday	

Exercise/ Cardio		
Monday		
Tuesday		
Wednesday		
Thursday		
Friday		
Saturday		
Sunday		

Specify whether Cardio or Strength Training. E/C

Weekly Menu

Monday:

Tuesday:

Wednesday:

Thursday:

Friday:

Weekend:

Saturday	Sunday

Put a check mark if you ate on time!	Brkfast		Lunch		Dinner	
Monday						
Tuesday	✓					
Wednesday						
Thursday						
Friday						
Saturday						
Sunday						

1 hr After each meal write an emoji for how you feel as far as energy, happy for good sad for bad!

Habit Tracker

Positive Pick New		Negative Pick Old	

Use The initials of each day to track Your New & Old Habits

Water Intake	64oz. 's
Monday	
Tuesday	
Wednesday	
Thursday	
Friday	
Saturday	
Sunday	

Exercise/ Cardio		
Monday		
Tuesday		
Wednesday		
Thursday		
Friday		
Saturday		
Sunday		

Specify whether Cardio or Strength Training. E/C

Weekly Menu

Monday:

Tuesday:

Wednesday:

Thursday:

Friday:

Weekend:

Saturday	Sunday

Put a check mark if you ate on time!	Brkfast	Lunch	Dinner
Monday			
Tuesday			
Wednesday			
Thursday			
Friday			
Saturday			
Sunday			

1 hr After each meal write an emoji for how you feel as far as energy, happy for good sad for bad!

Habit Tracker

Positive Pick New	Negative Pick Old

Use The initials of each day to track Your New & Old Habits

Water Intake	64oz. 's
Monday	
Tuesday	
Wednesday	
Thursday	
Friday	
Saturday	
Sunday	

Exercise/ Cardio		
Monday		
Tuesday		
Wednesday		
Thursday		
Friday		
Saturday		
Sunday		

Specify whether Cardio or Strength Training. E/C

Weekly Menu

Monday:

Tuesday:

Wednesday:

Thursday:

Friday:

Weekend:

Saturday	Sunday

Put a check mark if you ate on time!	Brkfast	Lunch	Dinner
Monday			
Tuesday	✓		
Wednesday			
Thursday			
Friday			
Saturday			
Sunday			

1 hr After each meal write an emoji for how you feel as far as energy, happy for good sad for bad!

Habit Tracker

Positive Pick New	Negative Pick Old

Use The initials of each day to track Your New & Old Habits

Water Intake	64oz. 's
Monday	
Tuesday	
Wednesday	
Thursday	
Friday	
Saturday	
Sunday	

Exercise/ Cardio		
Monday		
Tuesday		
Wednesday		
Thursday		
Friday		
Saturday		
Sunday		

Specify whether Cardio or Strength Training. E/C

Weekly Menu

Monday:

Tuesday:

Wednesday:

Thursday:

Friday:

Weekend:

Saturday	Sunday

February 2020

Sun	Mon	Tue	Wed	Thu	Fri	Sat
Things To-Do List Or Remember **1.** **2.**		28	29	30	31	1
2	3	4 **RosaParks**	5	6	7	8
9	10	11	12 **Lin.Bday**	13	14	15 **Susan B.**
16	17 **Was.Bday**	18	19	20	21	22
23	24	25	26 **Ash**	27	28	29

Monthly Overview/Notes

Put a check mark if you ate on time!	Brkfast		Lunch		Dinner		Habit Tracker	
							Positive **Pick New**	Negative **Pick Old**
Monday							T	
Tuesday	✓							
Wednesday							W	F
Thursday								
Friday								
Saturday								
Sunday								

1 hr After each meal write an emoji for how you feel as far as energy, happy for good sad for bad!

Use The initials of each day to track Your New & Old Habits

Water Intake	64oz. 's
Monday	
Tuesday	
Wednesday	
Thursday	
Friday	
Saturday	
Sunday	

Weekly Menu

Monday:

Tuesday:

Wednesday:

Thursday:

Friday:

Exercise/ Cardio		
Monday		
Tuesday		
Wednesday		
Thursday		
Friday		
Saturday		
Sunday		

Specify whether Cardio or Strength Training. E/C

Weekend:

Saturday	Sunday

What are some New foods you can try make a list?	Brkfast	Lunch	Dinner
Monday			
Tuesday			
Wednesday			
Thursday			
Friday			
Saturday			
Sunday			

1 hr After each meal mark how you feel as far as energy, with the New Foods from Your list !

New Habits

What are some New things that You would like to try?

1.
2.
3.

Okay Pick one & Track

M	T	W	Th	F	S	S

Put a check mark each day to track Your New Habit for the next 6 Weeks

Water Intake	64oz. 's
Week 1	
Week 2	
Week 3	
Week 4	
Week 5	

Has drinking the 64oz.'s been an issue? Are you sipping regularly throughout the day?

Exercise/ Cardio	E	C
Week 1		
Week 2		
Week 3		
Week 4		
Week 5		

Fill in how many hours You Trained for each week

Progress Assessment

1-10 How do I feel about my progress/surgery?

How many pounds have I lost?

How do I look in the mirror?

Do I like what I see so far?

What has been the hardest adjustment/s thus far?

What can I do to make this transition easier?

Who can I call or count on for support?

Put a check mark if you ate on time!	Brkfast		Lunch		Dinner	
Monday						
Tuesday						
Wednesday						
Thursday						
Friday						
Saturday						
Sunday						

1 hr After each meal write an emoji for how you feel as far as energy, happy for good sad for bad!

Habit Tracker

Positive Pick New		Negative Pick Old	

Use The initials of each day to track Your New & Old Habits

Water Intake	64oz. 's
Monday	
Tuesday	
Wednesday	
Thursday	
Friday	
Saturday	
Sunday	

Exercise/ Cardio		
Monday		
Tuesday		
Wednesday		
Thursday		
Friday		
Saturday		
Sunday		

Specify whether Cardio or Strength Training. E/C

Weekly Menu

Monday:

Tuesday:

Wednesday:

Thursday:

Friday:

Weekend:

Saturday	Sunday

Put a check mark if you ate on time!	Brkfast	Lunch	Dinner
Monday			
Tuesday	✓		
Wednesday			
Thursday			
Friday			
Saturday			
Sunday			

1 hr After each meal write an emoji for how you feel as far as energy, happy for good sad for bad!

Habit Tracker

Positive Pick New	Negative Pick Old

Use The initials of each day to track Your New & Old Habits

Water Intake	64oz. 's
Monday	
Tuesday	
Wednesday	
Thursday	
Friday	
Saturday	
Sunday	

Exercise/ Cardio	
Monday	
Tuesday	
Wednesday	
Thursday	
Friday	
Saturday	
Sunday	

Specify whether Cardio or Strength Training. E/C

Weekly Menu

Monday:

Tuesday:

Wednesday:

Thursday:

Friday:

Weekend:

Saturday	Sunday

Put a check mark if you ate on time!	Brkfast		Lunch		Dinner	
Monday						
Tuesday	✓					
Wednesday						
Thursday						
Friday						
Saturday						
Sunday						

1 hr After each meal write an emoji for how you feel as far as energy, happy for good sad for bad!

Habit Tracker

Positive Pick New		Negative Pick Old	

Use The initials of each day to track Your New & Old Habits

Water Intake	64oz. 's
Monday	
Tuesday	
Wednesday	
Thursday	
Friday	
Saturday	
Sunday	

Exercise/ Cardio		
Monday		
Tuesday		
Wednesday		
Thursday		
Friday		
Saturday		
Sunday		

Specify whether Cardio or Strength Training. E/C

Weekly Menu

Monday:

Tuesday:

Wednesday:

Thursday:

Friday:

Weekend:

Saturday	Sunday

March 2020

Sun	Mon	Tue	Wed	Thu	Fri	Sat
1	2	3	4	5	6	7
8	9	10 **Purim**	11	12	13	14
15	16	17 **St. Pat's**	18	19 **Equinox**	20	21
22	23	24	25	26	27	28
29	30	31	1	2	3	

Monthly Overview/Notes

Put a check mark if you ate on time!	Brkfast		Lunch		Dinner	
Monday						
Tuesday	✓					
Wednesday						
Thursday						
Friday						
Saturday						
Sunday						

1 hr After each meal write an emoji for how you feel as far as energy, happy for good sad for bad!

Habit Tracker

Positive Pick New		Negative Pick Old	

Use The initials of each day to track Your New & Old Habits

Water Intake	64oz. 's
Monday	
Tuesday	
Wednesday	
Thursday	
Friday	
Saturday	
Sunday	

Exercise/ Cardio		
Monday		
Tuesday		
Wednesday		
Thursday		
Friday		
Saturday		
Sunday		

Specify whether Cardio or Strength Training. E/C

Weekly Menu

Monday:

Tuesday:

Wednesday:

Thursday:

Friday:

Weekend:

Saturday	Sunday

Put a check mark if you ate on time!	Brkfast	Lunch	Dinner
Monday			
Tuesday	✓		
Wednesday			
Thursday			
Friday			
Saturday			
Sunday			

1 hr After each meal write an emoji for how you feel as far as energy, happy for good sad for bad!

Habit Tracker

	Positive Pick New		Negative Pick Old
	T		
W			F

Use The initials of each day to track Your New & Old Habits

Water Intake	64oz. 's
Monday	
Tuesday	
Wednesday	
Thursday	
Friday	
Saturday	
Sunday	

Exercise/ Cardio		
Monday		
Tuesday		
Wednesday		
Thursday		
Friday		
Saturday		
Sunday		

Specify whether Cardio or Strength Training. E/C

Weekly Menu

Monday:

Tuesday:

Wednesday:

Thursday:

Friday:

Weekend:

Saturday	Sunday

What are some New foods you can try make a list?	Brkfast	Lunch	Dinner
Monday			
Tuesday			
Wednesday			
Thursday			
Friday			
Saturday			
Sunday			

1 hr After each meal mark how you feel as far as energy, with the New Foods from Your list !

New Habits

What are some New things that You would like to try?

1.
2.
3.

Okay Pick one & Track

M	T	W	Th	F	S	S

Put a check mark each day to track Your New Habit for the next 6 Weeks

Water Intake	64oz. 's
Week 11	
Week 12	
Week 13	
Week 14	
Week 15	

Fill in how many 12oz. cups You drank each week

Exercise/ Cardio	E	C
Week 11		
Week 12		
Week 13		
Week 14		
Week 15		

Fill in how many hours You Trained for each week

Progress Assessment

1-10 How do I feel about my progress?

How many pounds have I lost?

How many inches have I lost?

How do I look in the mirror?

What size is my clothing now?

Have I bought new clothes yet?

How has my energy been lately?

How have my workouts been?

Is it easier to plan my meals?

Have I received any compliments lately?

What do I like most, the way I feel or look?

What is a new food/recipe that I've tried lately?

Have I met any new friends or likeminded people?

How has the journey been thus far?

Put a check mark if you ate on time!	Brkfast	Lunch	Dinner
Monday			
Tuesday	✓		
Wednesday			
Thursday			
Friday			
Saturday			
Sunday			

1 hr After each meal write an emoji for how you feel as far as energy, happy for good sad for bad!

Habit Tracker

Positive Pick New	Negative Pick Old

Use The initials of each day to track Your New & Old Habits

Water Intake 64oz. 's	
Monday	
Tuesday	
Wednesday	
Thursday	
Friday	
Saturday	
Sunday	

Exercise/ Cardio	
Monday	
Tuesday	
Wednesday	
Thursday	
Friday	
Saturday	
Sunday	

Specify whether Cardio or Strength Training. E/C

Weekly Menu

Monday:

Tuesday:

Wednesday:

Thursday:

Friday:

Weekend:

Saturday	Sunday

Put a check mark if you ate on time!	Brkfast		Lunch		Dinner	
Monday						
Tuesday	✓					
Wednesday						
Thursday						
Friday						
Saturday						
Sunday						

1 hr After each meal write an emoji for how you feel as far as energy, happy for good sad for bad!

Habit Tracker

Positive Pick New		Negative Pick Old

Use The initials of each day to track Your New & Old Habits

Water Intake	64oz. 's
Monday	
Tuesday	
Wednesday	
Thursday	
Friday	
Saturday	
Sunday	

Exercise/ Cardio		
Monday		
Tuesday		
Wednesday		
Thursday		
Friday		
Saturday		
Sunday		

Specify whether Cardio or Strength Training. E/C

Weekly Menu

Monday:

Tuesday:

Wednesday:

Thursday:

Friday:

Weekend:

Saturday	Sunday

Put a check mark if you ate on time!	Brkfast		Lunch		Dinner	
Monday						
Tuesday	✓					
Wednesday						
Thursday						
Friday						
Saturday						
Sunday						

1 hr After each meal write an emoji for how you feel as far as energy, happy for good sad for bad!

Habit Tracker

Positive Pick New		Negative Pick Old	
	T		
W			F

Use The initials of each day to track Your New & Old Habits

Water Intake	64oz. 's
Monday	
Tuesday	
Wednesday	
Thursday	
Friday	
Saturday	
Sunday	

Exercise/ Cardio		
Monday		
Tuesday		
Wednesday		
Thursday		
Friday		
Saturday		
Sunday		

Specify whether Cardio or Strength Training. E/C

Weekly Menu

Monday:

Tuesday:

Wednesday:

Thursday:

Friday:

Weekend:

Saturday	Sunday

April 2020

Sun	Mon	Tue	Wed	Thu	Fri	Sat
30	31	1	2	3	4	
5 Palm	6	7	8	9 PassOver	10 Good	11
12 Easter	13	14	15 TaxDay	16 LD/PasOv	17	18
19	20	21 Yom HaS.	22	23	24 Ramadan	25
26	27	28	29 Yom Ha'a	30	1	2

Monthly Overview/Notes

Put a check mark if you ate on time!	Brkfast		Lunch		Dinner	
Monday						
Tuesday						
Wednesday						
Thursday						
Friday						
Saturday						
Sunday						

1 hr After each meal write an emoji for how you feel as far as energy, happy for good sad for bad!

Habit Tracker

Positive Pick New	Negative Pick Old

Use The initials of each day to track Your New & Old Habits

Water Intake	64oz. 's
Monday	
Tuesday	
Wednesday	
Thursday	
Friday	
Saturday	
Sunday	

Exercise/ Cardio		
Monday		
Tuesday		
Wednesday		
Thursday		
Friday		
Saturday		
Sunday		

Specify whether Cardio or Strength Training. E/C

Weekly Menu

Monday:

Tuesday:

Wednesday:

Thursday:

Friday:

Weekend:

Saturday	Sunday

Put a check mark if you ate on time!	Brkfast		Lunch		Dinner	
Monday						
Tuesday	✓					
Wednesday						
Thursday						
Friday						
Saturday						
Sunday						

1 hr After each meal write an emoji for how you feel as far as energy, happy for good sad for bad!

Habit Tracker

Positive Pick New		Negative Pick Old	

Use The initials of each day to track Your New & Old Habits

Water Intake	64oz. 's
Monday	
Tuesday	
Wednesday	
Thursday	
Friday	
Saturday	
Sunday	

Exercise/ Cardio	
Monday	
Tuesday	
Wednesday	
Thursday	
Friday	
Saturday	
Sunday	

Specify whether Cardio or Strength Training. E/C

Weekly Menu

Monday:

Tuesday:

Wednesday:

Thursday:

Friday:

Weekend:

Saturday	Sunday

Put a check mark if you ate on time!	Brkfast	Lunch	Dinner
Monday			
Tuesday	✓		
Wednesday			
Thursday			
Friday			
Saturday			
Sunday			

1 hr After each meal write an emoji for how you feel as far as energy, happy for good sad for bad!

Habit Tracker

Positive Pick New	Negative Pick Old

Use The initials of each day to track Your New & Old Habits

Water Intake	64oz. 's
Monday	
Tuesday	
Wednesday	
Thursday	
Friday	
Saturday	
Sunday	

Weekly Menu

Monday:

Tuesday:

Wednesday:

Thursday:

Friday:

Weekend:

Saturday	Sunday

Exercise/ Cardio	
Monday	
Tuesday	
Wednesday	
Thursday	
Friday	
Saturday	
Sunday	

Specify whether Cardio or Strength Training. E/C

Put a check mark if you ate on time!	Brkfast		Lunch		Dinner	
Monday						
Tuesday						
Wednesday						
Thursday						
Friday						
Saturday						
Sunday						

1 hr After each meal write an emoji for how you feel as far as energy, happy for good sad for bad!

Habit Tracker

Positive Pick New		Negative Pick Old	

Use The initials of each day to track Your New & Old Habits

Water Intake	64oz. 's
Monday	
Tuesday	
Wednesday	
Thursday	
Friday	
Saturday	
Sunday	

Weekly Menu

Monday:

Tuesday:

Wednesday:

Thursday:

Friday:

Weekend:

Saturday	Sunday

Exercise/ Cardio		
Monday		
Tuesday		
Wednesday		
Thursday		
Friday		
Saturday		
Sunday		

Specify whether Cardio or Strength Training. E/C

Put a check mark if you ate on time!	Brkfast	Lunch	Dinner
Monday			
Tuesday	✓		
Wednesday			
Thursday			
Friday			
Saturday			
Sunday			

1 hr After each meal write an emoji for how you feel as far as energy, happy for good sad for bad!

Habit Tracker

Positive Pick New	Negative Pick Old

Use The initials of each day to track Your New & Old Habits

Water Intake 64oz. 's	
Monday	
Tuesday	
Wednesday	
Thursday	
Friday	
Saturday	
Sunday	

Exercise/ Cardio		
Monday		
Tuesday		
Wednesday		
Thursday		
Friday		
Saturday		
Sunday		

Specify whether Cardio or Strength Training. E/C

Weekly Menu

Monday:

Tuesday:

Wednesday:

Thursday:

Friday:

Weekend:

Saturday	Sunday

May 2020

Sun	Mon	Tue	Wed	Thu	Fri	Sat
27	28	29	30	1	2	
3	4	5 Cinco de	6	7	8	9
10 Mother's	11	12 Lag BaO	13	14	15	16
17	18	19	20	21	22	23
24	25 Memorial	26	27	28	29 Shavuot	30
31	1	2	3	4	5	6

Monthly Overview/Notes

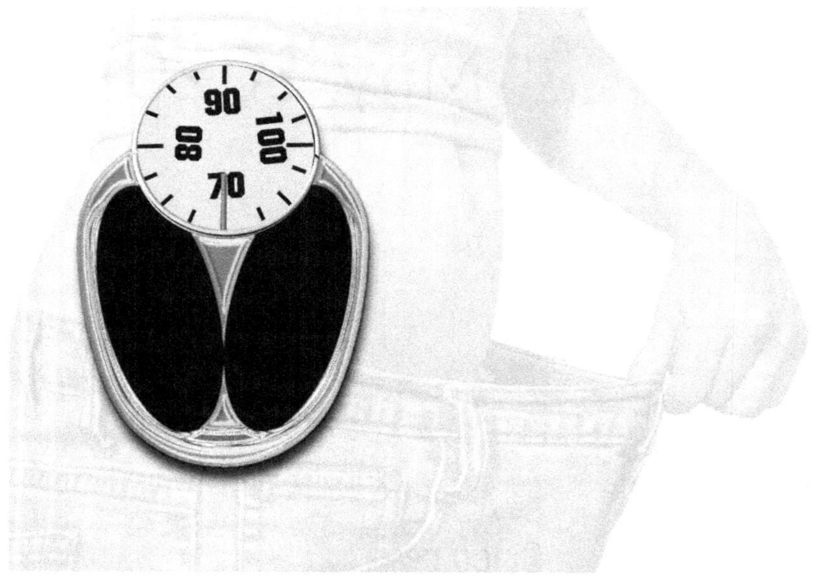

Measurements

Weight		Body Mass Index (BMI)	
Body Fat %		Water Weight	
Bust		Muscle Weight	
Chest		**Notes**	
Waist			
Hips			
Thighs			
Calves			
Upper Arm			
Fore Arm			

Well how is it going?????

How do you feel Overall?

Are you happy with your progress so far?

What have you cut out? Are you seeing more results?

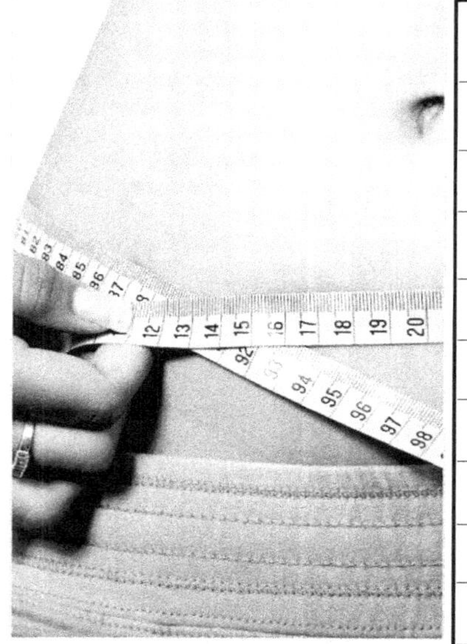

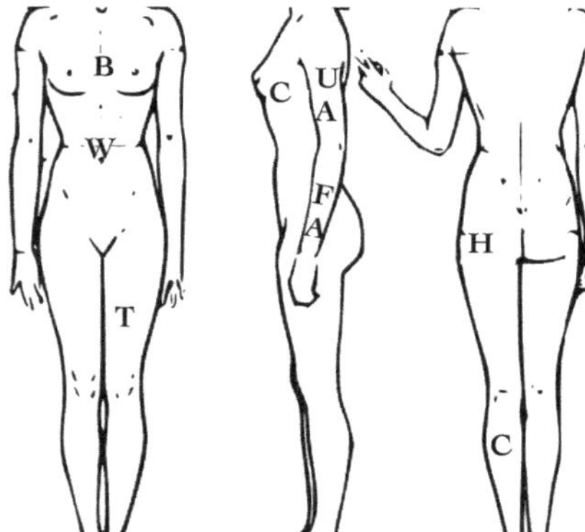

Put a check mark if you ate on time!	Brkfast	Lunch	Dinner
Monday			
Tuesday	✓		
Wednesday			
Thursday			
Friday			
Saturday			
Sunday			

1 hr After each meal write an emoji for how you feel as far as energy, happy for good sad for bad!

Habit Tracker

Positive Pick New		Negative Pick Old	

Use The initials of each day to track Your New & Old Habits

Water Intake	64oz. 's
Monday	
Tuesday	
Wednesday	
Thursday	
Friday	
Saturday	
Sunday	

Exercise/ Cardio		
Monday		
Tuesday		
Wednesday		
Thursday		
Friday		
Saturday		
Sunday		

Specify whether Cardio or Strength Training. E/C

Weekly Menu

Monday:

Tuesday:

Wednesday:

Thursday:

Friday:

Weekend:

Saturday	Sunday

Put a check mark if you ate on time!	Brkfast	Lunch	Dinner
Monday			
Tuesday			
Wednesday			
Thursday			
Friday			
Saturday			
Sunday			

1 hr After each meal write an emoji for how you feel as far as energy, happy for good sad for bad!

Habit Tracker

Positive Pick New	Negative Pick Old

Use The initials of each day to track Your New & Old Habits

Water Intake	64oz. 's
Monday	
Tuesday	
Wednesday	
Thursday	
Friday	
Saturday	
Sunday	

Weekly Menu

Monday:

Tuesday:

Wednesday:

Thursday:

Friday:

Exercise/ Cardio		
Monday		
Tuesday		
Wednesday		
Thursday		
Friday		
Saturday		
Sunday		

Specify whether Cardio or Strength Training. E/C

Weekend:

Saturday	Sunday

Put a check mark if you ate on time!	Brkfast	Lunch	Dinner
Monday			
Tuesday			
Wednesday			
Thursday			
Friday			
Saturday			
Sunday			

1 hr After each meal write an emoji for how you feel as far as energy, happy for good sad for bad!

Habit Tracker

Positive Pick New		Negative Pick Old	

Use The initials of each day to track Your New & Old Habits

Water Intake	64oz. 's
Monday	
Tuesday	
Wednesday	
Thursday	
Friday	
Saturday	
Sunday	

Exercise/ Cardio		
Monday		
Tuesday		
Wednesday		
Thursday		
Friday		
Saturday		
Sunday		

Specify whether Cardio or Strength Training. E/C

Weekly Menu

Monday:

Tuesday:

Wednesday:

Thursday:

Friday:

Weekend:

Saturday	Sunday

Put a check mark if you ate on time!	Brkfast	Lunch	Dinner
Monday			
Tuesday	✓		
Wednesday			
Thursday			
Friday			
Saturday			
Sunday			

1 hr After each meal write an emoji for how you feel as far as energy, happy for good sad for bad!

Habit Tracker

Positive Pick New	Negative Pick Old

Use The initials of each day to track Your New & Old Habits

Water Intake	64oz. 's
Monday	
Tuesday	
Wednesday	
Thursday	
Friday	
Saturday	
Sunday	

Weekly Menu

Monday:

Tuesday:

Wednesday:

Thursday:

Friday:

Weekend:

Saturday	Sunday

Exercise/ Cardio	
Monday	
Tuesday	
Wednesday	
Thursday	
Friday	
Saturday	
Sunday	

Specify whether Cardio or Strength Training. E/C

Put a check mark if you ate on time!	Brkfast		Lunch		Dinner	
Monday						
Tuesday						
Wednesday						
Thursday						
Friday						
Saturday						
Sunday						

1 hr After each meal write an emoji for how you feel as far as energy, happy for good sad for bad!

Habit Tracker

Positive Pick New		Negative Pick Old	

Use The initials of each day to track Your New & Old Habits

Water Intake	64oz. 's
Monday	
Tuesday	
Wednesday	
Thursday	
Friday	
Saturday	
Sunday	

Exercise/ Cardio		
Monday		
Tuesday		
Wednesday		
Thursday		
Friday		
Saturday		
Sunday		

Specify whether Cardio or Strength Training. E/C

Weekly Menu

Monday:

Tuesday:

Wednesday:

Thursday:

Friday:

Weekend:

Saturday	Sunday

June 2020

Sun	Mon	Tue	Wed	Thu	Fri	Sat
	1	2	3	4	5	6
7	8	9	10	11	12	13
14 Army	15	16	17	18	19 Teenth	20 Solstice
21 Father's	22	23	24	25	26	27
28	29	30	1	2	3	4

Monthly Overview/Notes

Put a check mark if you ate on time!	Brkfast	Lunch	Dinner
Monday			
Tuesday	✓		
Wednesday			
Thursday			
Friday			
Saturday			
Sunday			

1 hr After each meal write an emoji for how you feel as far as energy, happy for good sad for bad!

Habit Tracker

Positive Pick New		Negative Pick Old	

Use The initials of each day to track Your New & Old Habits

Water Intake	64oz. 's
Monday	
Tuesday	
Wednesday	
Thursday	
Friday	
Saturday	
Sunday	

Weekly Menu

Monday:

Tuesday:

Wednesday:

Thursday:

Friday:

Exercise/ Cardio		
Monday		
Tuesday		
Wednesday		
Thursday		
Friday		
Saturday		
Sunday		

Specify whether Cardio or Strength Training. E/C

Weekend:

Saturday	Sunday

Put a check mark if you ate on time!	Brkfast	Lunch	Dinner
Monday			
Tuesday	✓		
Wednesday			
Thursday			
Friday			
Saturday			
Sunday			

1 hr After each meal write an emoji for how you feel as far as energy, happy for good sad for bad!

Habit Tracker

Positive Pick New	Negative Pick Old

Use The initials of each day to track Your New & Old Habits

Water Intake	64oz. 's
Monday	
Tuesday	
Wednesday	
Thursday	
Friday	
Saturday	
Sunday	

Exercise/ Cardio	
Monday	
Tuesday	
Wednesday	
Thursday	
Friday	
Saturday	
Sunday	

Specify whether Cardio or Strength Training. E/C

Weekly Menu

Monday:

Tuesday:

Wednesday:

Thursday:

Friday:

Weekend:

Saturday	Sunday

<table>
<tr><td>Put a check mark if you ate on time!</td><td>Brkfast</td><td>Lunch</td><td>Dinner</td></tr>
<tr><td>Monday</td><td></td><td></td><td></td></tr>
<tr><td>Tuesday</td><td></td><td></td><td></td></tr>
<tr><td>Wednesday</td><td></td><td></td><td></td></tr>
<tr><td>Thursday</td><td></td><td></td><td></td></tr>
<tr><td>Friday</td><td></td><td></td><td></td></tr>
<tr><td>Saturday</td><td></td><td></td><td></td></tr>
<tr><td>Sunday</td><td></td><td></td><td></td></tr>
</table>

1 hr After each meal write an emoji for how you feel as far as energy, happy for good sad for bad!

Habit Tracker

Positive Pick New	Negative Pick Old

Use The initials of each day to track Your New & Old Habits

Water Intake	64oz. 's
Monday	
Tuesday	
Wednesday	
Thursday	
Friday	
Saturday	
Sunday	

Exercise/ Cardio		
Monday		
Tuesday		
Wednesday		
Thursday		
Friday		
Saturday		
Sunday		

Specify whether Cardio or Strength Training. E/C

Weekly Menu

Monday:

Tuesday:

Wednesday:

Thursday:

Friday:

Weekend:

Saturday	Sunday

Put a check mark if you ate on time!	Brkfast	Lunch	Dinner
Monday			
Tuesday	✓		
Wednesday			
Thursday			
Friday			
Saturday			
Sunday			

1 hr After each meal write an emoji for how you feel as far as energy, happy for good sad for bad!

Habit Tracker

Positive **Pick New**	Negative **Pick Old**

Use The initials of each day to track Your New & Old Habits

Water Intake	64oz. 's
Monday	
Tuesday	
Wednesday	
Thursday	
Friday	
Saturday	
Sunday	

Weekly Menu

Monday:

Tuesday:

Wednesday:

Thursday:

Friday:

Exercise/ Cardio	
Monday	
Tuesday	
Wednesday	
Thursday	
Friday	
Saturday	
Sunday	

Specify whether Cardio or Strength Training. E/C

Weekend:	
Saturday	Sunday

July 2020

Sun	Mon	Tue	Wed	Thu	Fri	Sat
	29	30	1	2	3	4 **Indepen.**
5	6	7	8	9	10	11
12	13	14	15	16	17	18
19	20	21	22	23	24	25
26	27	28	29	30 **TishaB'Av**	31	1

Monthly Overview/Notes

Put a check mark if you ate on time!	Brkfast		Lunch		Dinner	
Monday						
Tuesday	✓					
Wednesday						
Thursday						
Friday						
Saturday						
Sunday						

1 hr After each meal write an emoji for how you feel as far as energy, happy for good sad for bad!

Habit Tracker

Positive Pick New	Negative Pick Old

Use The initials of each day to track Your New & Old Habits

Water Intake	64oz. 's
Monday	
Tuesday	
Wednesday	
Thursday	
Friday	
Saturday	
Sunday	

Exercise/ Cardio	
Monday	
Tuesday	
Wednesday	
Thursday	
Friday	
Saturday	
Sunday	

Specify whether Cardio or Strength Training. E/C

Weekly Menu

Monday:

Tuesday:

Wednesday:

Thursday:

Friday:

Weekend:

Saturday	Sunday

Put a check mark if you ate on time!	Brkfast		Lunch		Dinner	
Monday						
Tuesday						
Wednesday						
Thursday						
Friday						
Saturday						
Sunday						

1 hr After each meal write an emoji for how you feel as far as energy, happy for good sad for bad!

Habit Tracker

Positive Pick New		Negative Pick Old	

Use The initials of each day to track Your New & Old Habits

Water Intake	64oz. 's
Monday	
Tuesday	
Wednesday	
Thursday	
Friday	
Saturday	
Sunday	

Exercise/ Cardio	
Monday	
Tuesday	
Wednesday	
Thursday	
Friday	
Saturday	
Sunday	

Specify whether Cardio or Strength Training. E/C

Weekly Menu

Monday:

Tuesday:

Wednesday:

Thursday:

Friday:

Weekend:

Saturday	Sunday

Put a check mark if you ate on time!	Brkfast	Lunch	Dinner
Monday			
Tuesday			
Wednesday			
Thursday			
Friday			
Saturday			
Sunday			

1 hr After each meal write an emoji for how you feel as far as energy, happy for good sad for bad!

Habit Tracker

Positive Pick New	Negative Pick Old

Use The initials of each day to track Your New & Old Habits

Water Intake	64oz. 's
Monday	
Tuesday	
Wednesday	
Thursday	
Friday	
Saturday	
Sunday	

Exercise/ Cardio	
Monday	
Tuesday	
Wednesday	
Thursday	
Friday	
Saturday	
Sunday	

Specify whether Cardio or Strength Training. E/C

Weekly Menu

Monday:

Tuesday:

Wednesday:

Thursday:

Friday:

Weekend:

Saturday	Sunday

Put a check mark if you ate on time!	Brkfast	Lunch	Dinner
Monday			
Tuesday			
Wednesday			
Thursday			
Friday			
Saturday			
Sunday			

1 hr After each meal write an emoji for how you feel as far as energy, happy for good sad for bad!

Habit Tracker

Positive Pick New	Negative Pick Old

Use The initials of each day to track Your New & Old Habits

Water Intake	64oz. 's
Monday	
Tuesday	
Wednesday	
Thursday	
Friday	
Saturday	
Sunday	

Exercise/ Cardio		
Monday		
Tuesday		
Wednesday		
Thursday		
Friday		
Saturday		
Sunday		

Specify whether Cardio or Strength Training. E/C

Weekly Menu

Monday:

Tuesday:

Wednesday:

Thursday:

Friday:

Weekend:

Saturday	Sunday

Put a check mark if you ate on time!	Brkfast	Lunch	Dinner
Monday			
Tuesday	✓		
Wednesday			
Thursday			
Friday			
Saturday			
Sunday			

1 hr After each meal write an emoji for how you feel as far as energy, happy for good sad for bad!

Habit Tracker

Positive Pick New	Negative Pick Old

Use The initials of each day to track Your New & Old Habits

Water Intake	64oz. 's
Monday	
Tuesday	
Wednesday	
Thursday	
Friday	
Saturday	
Sunday	

Exercise/ Cardio		
Monday		
Tuesday		
Wednesday		
Thursday		
Friday		
Saturday		
Sunday		

Specify whether Cardio or Strength Training. E/C

Weekly Menu

Monday:

Tuesday:

Wednesday:

Thursday:

Friday:

Weekend:

Saturday	Sunday

August 2020

Sun	Mon	Tue	Wed	Thu	Fri	Sat
	27	28	29	30	31	1
2	3	4	5	6	7	8
9	10	11	12	13	14	15
16	17	18	19	20	21	22
23	24	25	26	27	28	29
30	31	1	2	3	4	5

Monthly Overview/Notes

Put a check mark if you ate on time!	Brkfast		Lunch		Dinner	
Monday						
Tuesday	✓					
Wednesday						
Thursday						
Friday						
Saturday						
Sunday						

🎭 1 hr After each meal write an emoji for how you feel as far as energy, happy for good sad for bad!

Habit Tracker

Positive Pick New		Negative Pick Old

Use The initials of each day to track Your New & Old Habits

Water Intake	64oz. 🥤's
Monday	
Tuesday	
Wednesday	
Thursday	
Friday	
Saturday	
Sunday	

Weekly Menu

Monday:

Tuesday:

Wednesday:

Thursday:

Friday:

Weekend:

Saturday	Sunday

Exercise/ Cardio 🏋🏃	🕐
Monday	
Tuesday	
Wednesday	
Thursday	
Friday	
Saturday	
Sunday	

Specify whether Cardio or Strength Training. E/C

Put a check mark if you ate on time!	Brkfast	Lunch	Dinner
Monday			
Tuesday	✓		
Wednesday			
Thursday			
Friday			
Saturday			
Sunday			

1 hr After each meal write an emoji for how you feel as far as energy, happy for good sad for bad!

Habit Tracker

Positive Pick New	Negative Pick Old

Use The initials of each day to track Your New & Old Habits

Water Intake	64oz. 's
Monday	
Tuesday	
Wednesday	
Thursday	
Friday	
Saturday	
Sunday	

Exercise/ Cardio	
Monday	
Tuesday	
Wednesday	
Thursday	
Friday	
Saturday	
Sunday	

Specify whether Cardio or Strength Training. E/C

Weekly Menu

Monday:

Tuesday:

Wednesday:

Thursday:

Friday:

Weekend:

Saturday	Sunday

What are some New foods you can try make a list?	Brkfast	Lunch	Dinner
Monday			
Tuesday			
Wednesday			
Thursday			
Friday			
Saturday			
Sunday			

1 hr After each meal mark how you feel as far as energy, with the New Foods from Your list !

New Habits

What are some New things that You would like to try?

1.
2.
3.

Okay Pick one & Track

M	T	W	Th	F	S	S

Put a check mark each day to track Your New Habit for the next 6 Weeks

Water Intake	64oz. 's
Week 35	
Week 36	
Week 37	
Week 38	
Week 39	

Did you drink at least 64 oz. of water every day each week?

Exercise/ Cardio	E	C
Week 35		
Week 36		
Week 37		
Week 38		
Week 39		

Fill in how many hours You Trained for each week

Progress Assessment

1-10 How do I feel about my progress?

How many pounds have I lost?

How many inches have I lost?

How do I look in the mirror?

What size is my clothing now?

Have I bought new clothes yet?

How has my energy been lately?

How have my workouts been?

How have you been in regards to health?

What do you like most, the way you feel or look? Why?

What do I enjoy most, exercise or eating healthy?

Who is one person that you can support to get healthy?

Who do you need to stay away from & Why?

Put a check mark if you ate on time!	Brkfast	Lunch	Dinner
Monday			
Tuesday	✓		
Wednesday			
Thursday			
Friday			
Saturday			
Sunday			

1 hr After each meal write an emoji for how you feel as far as energy, happy for good sad for bad!

Habit Tracker

Positive Pick New	Negative Pick Old

Use The initials of each day to track Your New & Old Habits

Water Intake	64oz. 's
Monday	
Tuesday	
Wednesday	
Thursday	
Friday	
Saturday	
Sunday	

Exercise/ Cardio	
Monday	
Tuesday	
Wednesday	
Thursday	
Friday	
Saturday	
Sunday	

Specify whether Cardio or Strength Training. E/C

Weekly Menu

Monday:

Tuesday:

Wednesday:

Thursday:

Friday:

Weekend:

Saturday	Sunday

Put a check mark if you ate on time!	Brkfast		Lunch		Dinner	
Monday						
Tuesday						
Wednesday						
Thursday						
Friday						
Saturday						
Sunday						

1 hr After each meal write an emoji for how you feel as far as energy, happy for good sad for bad!

Habit Tracker

Positive Pick New	Negative Pick Old
T	
W	F

Use The initials of each day to track Your New & Old Habits

Water Intake	64oz. 's
Monday	
Tuesday	
Wednesday	
Thursday	
Friday	
Saturday	
Sunday	

Weekly Menu

Monday:

Tuesday:

Wednesday:

Thursday:

Friday:

Exercise/ Cardio		
Monday		
Tuesday		
Wednesday		
Thursday		
Friday		
Saturday		
Sunday		

Specify whether Cardio or Strength Training. E/C

Weekend:

Saturday	Sunday

<table>
<tr><td>

Put a check mark if you ate on time!	Brkfast		Lunch		Dinner	
Monday						
Tuesday						
Wednesday						
Thursday						
Friday						
Saturday						
Sunday						

1 hr After each meal write an emoji for how you feel as far as energy, happy for good sad for bad!

</td><td>

Habit Tracker

Positive Pick New		Negative Pick Old	

Use The initials of each day to track Your New & Old Habits

</td></tr>
</table>

Water Intake	64oz. 's
Monday	
Tuesday	
Wednesday	
Thursday	
Friday	
Saturday	
Sunday	

Exercise/ Cardio		
Monday		
Tuesday		
Wednesday		
Thursday		
Friday		
Saturday		
Sunday		

Specify whether Cardio or Strength Training. E/C

Weekly Menu

Monday:

Tuesday:

Wednesday:

Thursday:

Friday:

Weekend:

Saturday	Sunday

September 2020

Sun	Mon	Tue	Wed	Thu	Fri	Sat
	31	1	2	3	4	5
6	7 Labor	8	9	10	11	12
13	14	15	16	17	18 Air Force	19 Rosh Has.
20	21	22	23	24	25	26
27	28 Yom Kip.	29	30	1	2	3

Monthly Overview/Notes

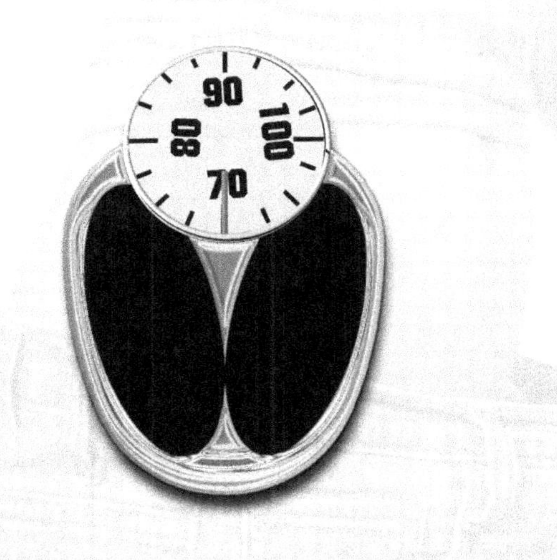

Measurements

Weight		Body Mass Index (BMI)	
Body Fat %		Water Weight	
Bust		Muscle Weight	
Chest		**Notes**	
Waist			
Hips			
Thighs			
Calves			
Upper Arm			
Fore Arm			

Do you notice anything new energy, feelings, etc?

Ok it's been a while how faithful have you been?

Are you happy with your progress so far?

Have you been loving or neglecting yourself??? Why?

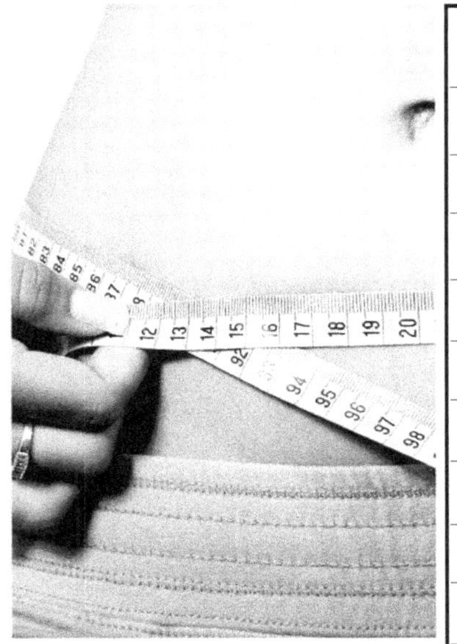

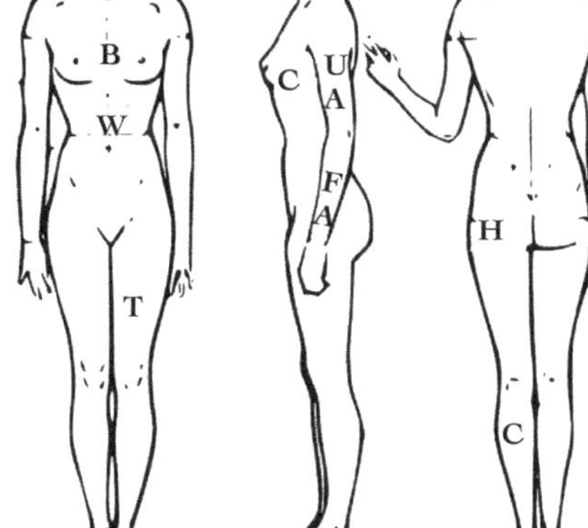

Put a check mark if you ate on time!	Brkfast		Lunch		Dinner	
Monday						
Tuesday	✓					
Wednesday						
Thursday						
Friday						
Saturday						
Sunday						

1 hr After each meal write an emoji for how you feel as far as energy, happy for good sad for bad!

Habit Tracker

Positive Pick New	Negative Pick Old

Use The initials of each day to track Your New & Old Habits

Water Intake	64oz. 's
Monday	
Tuesday	
Wednesday	
Thursday	
Friday	
Saturday	
Sunday	

Exercise/ Cardio		
Monday		
Tuesday		
Wednesday		
Thursday		
Friday		
Saturday		
Sunday		

Specify whether Cardio or Strength Training. E/C

Weekly Menu

Monday:

Tuesday:

Wednesday:

Thursday:

Friday:

Weekend:

Saturday	Sunday

Put a check mark if you ate on time!	Brkfast		Lunch		Dinner	
Monday						
Tuesday	✓					
Wednesday						
Thursday						
Friday						
Saturday						
Sunday						

1 hr After each meal write an emoji for how you feel as far as energy, happy for good sad for bad!

Habit Tracker

Positive Pick New	Negative Pick Old

Use The initials of each day to track Your New & Old Habits

Water Intake	64oz. 's
Monday	
Tuesday	
Wednesday	
Thursday	
Friday	
Saturday	
Sunday	

Exercise/ Cardio		
Monday		
Tuesday		
Wednesday		
Thursday		
Friday		
Saturday		
Sunday		

Specify whether Cardio or Strength Training. E/C

Weekly Menu

Monday:

Tuesday:

Wednesday:

Thursday:

Friday:

Weekend:

Saturday	Sunday

Put a check mark if you ate on time!	Brkfast		Lunch		Dinner	
Monday						
Tuesday						
Wednesday						
Thursday						
Friday						
Saturday						
Sunday						

1 hr After each meal write an emoji for how you feel as far as energy, happy for good sad for bad!

Habit Tracker

Positive Pick New		Negative Pick Old	
	T		
W			F

Use The initials of each day to track Your New & Old Habits

Water Intake	64oz. 's
Monday	
Tuesday	
Wednesday	
Thursday	
Friday	
Saturday	
Sunday	

Exercise/ Cardio		
Monday		
Tuesday		
Wednesday		
Thursday		
Friday		
Saturday		
Sunday		

Specify whether Cardio or Strength Training. E/C

Weekly Menu

Monday:

Tuesday:

Wednesday:

Thursday:

Friday:

Weekend:

Saturday	Sunday

Put a check mark if you ate on time!	Brkfast		Lunch		Dinner	
Monday						
Tuesday	✓					
Wednesday						
Thursday						
Friday						
Saturday						
Sunday						

1 hr After each meal write an emoji for how you feel as far as energy, happy for good sad for bad!

Habit Tracker

Positive Pick New	Negative Pick Old

Use The initials of each day to track Your New & Old Habits

Water Intake	64oz. 's
Monday	
Tuesday	
Wednesday	
Thursday	
Friday	
Saturday	
Sunday	

Exercise/ Cardio		
Monday		
Tuesday		
Wednesday		
Thursday		
Friday		
Saturday		
Sunday		

Specify whether Cardio or Strength Training. E/C

Weekly Menu

Monday:

Tuesday:

Wednesday:

Thursday:

Friday:

Weekend:

Saturday	Sunday

Put a check mark if you ate on time!	Brkfast	Lunch	Dinner
Monday			
Tuesday	✓		
Wednesday			
Thursday			
Friday			
Saturday			
Sunday			

1 hr After each meal write an emoji for how you feel as far as energy, happy for good sad for bad!

Habit Tracker

Positive Pick New	Negative Pick Old

Use The initials of each day to track Your New & Old Habits

Water Intake	64oz. 's
Monday	
Tuesday	
Wednesday	
Thursday	
Friday	
Saturday	
Sunday	

Exercise/ Cardio		
Monday		
Tuesday		
Wednesday		
Thursday		
Friday		
Saturday		
Sunday		

Specify whether Cardio or Strength Training. E/C

Weekly Menu

Monday:

Tuesday:

Wednesday:

Thursday:

Friday:

Weekend:

Saturday	Sunday

October 2020

Sun	Mon	Tue	Wed	Thu	Fri	Sat
28	29	30	1	2	3 1st. D Suk
4	5	6	7	8	9 Last Suk.	10 Shm.Atz
11 Sim.Tor	12 Columbus	13 Navy	14	15	16	17
18	19	20	21	22	23	24
25	26	27	28	29	30	31 Halloween

Monthly Overview/Notes

Put a check mark if you ate on time!	Brkfast	Lunch	Dinner
Monday			
Tuesday			
Wednesday			
Thursday			
Friday			
Saturday			
Sunday			

1 hr After each meal write an emoji for how you feel as far as energy, happy for good sad for bad!

Habit Tracker

Positive Pick New	Negative Pick Old

Use The initials of each day to track Your New & Old Habits

Water Intake	64oz. 's
Monday	
Tuesday	
Wednesday	
Thursday	
Friday	
Saturday	
Sunday	

Exercise/ Cardio	
Monday	
Tuesday	
Wednesday	
Thursday	
Friday	
Saturday	
Sunday	

Specify whether Cardio or Strength Training. E/C

Weekly Menu

Monday:

Tuesday:

Wednesday:

Thursday:

Friday:

Weekend:

Saturday	Sunday

Put a check mark if you ate on time!	Brkfast	Lunch	Dinner
Monday			
Tuesday			
Wednesday			
Thursday			
Friday			
Saturday			
Sunday			

1 hr After each meal write an emoji for how you feel as far as energy, happy for good sad for bad!

Habit Tracker

	Positive Pick New		Negative Pick Old

Use The initials of each day to track Your New & Old Habits

Water Intake	64oz. 's
Monday	
Tuesday	
Wednesday	
Thursday	
Friday	
Saturday	
Sunday	

Exercise/ Cardio	
Monday	
Tuesday	
Wednesday	
Thursday	
Friday	
Saturday	
Sunday	

Specify whether Cardio or Strength Training. E/C

Weekly Menu

Monday:

Tuesday:

Wednesday:

Thursday:

Friday:

Weekend:

Saturday	Sunday

Put a check mark if you ate on time!	Brkfast		Lunch		Dinner	
Monday						
Tuesday	✓					
Wednesday						
Thursday						
Friday						
Saturday						
Sunday						

1 hr After each meal write an emoji for how you feel as far as energy, happy for good sad for bad!

Habit Tracker

Positive Pick New	Negative Pick Old

Use The initials of each day to track Your New & Old Habits

Water Intake	64oz. 's
Monday	
Tuesday	
Wednesday	
Thursday	
Friday	
Saturday	
Sunday	

Weekly Menu

Monday:

Tuesday:

Wednesday:

Thursday:

Friday:

Weekend:

Saturday	Sunday

Exercise/ Cardio	
Monday	
Tuesday	
Wednesday	
Thursday	
Friday	
Saturday	
Sunday	

Specify whether Cardio or Strength Training. E/C

Put a check mark if you ate on time!	Brkfast	Lunch	Dinner
Monday			
Tuesday	✓		
Wednesday			
Thursday			
Friday			
Saturday			
Sunday			

1 hr After each meal write an emoji for how you feel as far as energy, happy for good sad for bad!

Habit Tracker

Positive Pick New	Negative Pick Old

Use The initials of each day to track Your New & Old Habits

Water Intake	64oz. 's
Monday	
Tuesday	
Wednesday	
Thursday	
Friday	
Saturday	
Sunday	

Exercise/ Cardio		
Monday		
Tuesday		
Wednesday		
Thursday		
Friday		
Saturday		
Sunday		

Specify whether Cardio or Strength Training. E/C

Weekly Menu

Monday:

Tuesday:

Wednesday:

Thursday:

Friday:

Weekend:

Saturday	Sunday

Put a check mark if you ate on time!	Brkfast	Lunch	Dinner
Monday			
Tuesday			
Wednesday			
Thursday			
Friday			
Saturday			
Sunday			

1 hr After each meal write an emoji for how you feel as far as energy, happy for good sad for bad!

Habit Tracker

Positive Pick New	Negative Pick Old

Use The initials of each day to track Your New & Old Habits

Water Intake	64oz. 's
Monday	
Tuesday	
Wednesday	
Thursday	
Friday	
Saturday	
Sunday	

Exercise/ Cardio		
Monday		
Tuesday		
Wednesday		
Thursday		
Friday		
Saturday		
Sunday		

Specify whether Cardio or Strength Training. E/C

Weekly Menu

Monday:

Tuesday:

Wednesday:

Thursday:

Friday:

Weekend:

Saturday	Sunday

November 2020

Sun	Mon	Tue	Wed	Thu	Fri	Sat
1 **DLS**	2	3 **Election**	4	5	6	7
8	9	10	11 **Veterans**	12	13	14
15	16	17	18	19	20	21
22	23	24	25	26 **Thanks Giving**	27 **Black Friday**	28
29	30 **Cyber Monday**	1	2	3	4	

Monthly Overview/Notes

<table>
<tr><td>Put a check mark if you ate on time!</td><td>Brkfast</td><td>Lunch</td><td>Dinner</td></tr>
<tr><td>Monday</td><td></td><td></td><td></td></tr>
<tr><td>Tuesday</td><td>✓</td><td></td><td></td></tr>
<tr><td>Wednesday</td><td></td><td></td><td></td></tr>
<tr><td>Thursday</td><td></td><td></td><td></td></tr>
<tr><td>Friday</td><td></td><td></td><td></td></tr>
<tr><td>Saturday</td><td></td><td></td><td></td></tr>
<tr><td>Sunday</td><td></td><td></td><td></td></tr>
</table>

1 hr After each meal write an emoji for how you feel as far as energy, happy for good sad for bad!

Habit Tracker

Positive Pick New	Negative Pick Old
T	
W	F

Use The initials of each day to track Your New & Old Habits

Water Intake	64oz. 's
Monday	
Tuesday	
Wednesday	
Thursday	
Friday	
Saturday	
Sunday	

Exercise/ Cardio		
Monday		
Tuesday		
Wednesday		
Thursday		
Friday		
Saturday		
Sunday		

Specify whether Cardio or Strength Training. E/C

Weekly Menu

Monday:

Tuesday:

Wednesday:

Thursday:

Friday:

Weekend:

Saturday	Sunday

Put a check mark if you ate on time!	Brkfast		Lunch		Dinner	
Monday						
Tuesday						
Wednesday						
Thursday						
Friday						
Saturday						
Sunday						

1 hr After each meal write an emoji for how you feel as far as energy, happy for good sad for bad!

Habit Tracker

Positive Pick New	Negative Pick Old

Use The initials of each day to track Your New & Old Habits

Water Intake	64oz. 's
Monday	
Tuesday	
Wednesday	
Thursday	
Friday	
Saturday	
Sunday	

Exercise/ Cardio		
Monday		
Tuesday		
Wednesday		
Thursday		
Friday		
Saturday		
Sunday		

Specify whether Cardio or Strength Training. E/C

Weekly Menu

Monday:

Tuesday:

Wednesday:

Thursday:

Friday:

Weekend:

Saturday	Sunday

Put a check mark if you ate on time!	Brkfast	Lunch	Dinner
Monday			
Tuesday			
Wednesday			
Thursday			
Friday			
Saturday			
Sunday			

1 hr After each meal write an emoji for how you feel as far as energy, happy for good sad for bad!

Habit Tracker

Positive Pick New	Negative Pick Old

Use The initials of each day to track Your New & Old Habits

Water Intake	64oz. 's
Monday	
Tuesday	
Wednesday	
Thursday	
Friday	
Saturday	
Sunday	

Weekly Menu

Monday:

Tuesday:

Wednesday:

Thursday:

Friday:

Weekend:

Saturday	Sunday

Exercise/ Cardio		
Monday		
Tuesday		
Wednesday		
Thursday		
Friday		
Saturday		
Sunday		

Specify whether Cardio or Strength Training. E/C

Put a check mark if you ate on time!	Brkfast		Lunch		Dinner	
Monday						
Tuesday	✓					
Wednesday						
Thursday						
Friday						
Saturday						
Sunday						

1 hr After each meal write an emoji for how you feel as far as energy, happy for good sad for bad!

Habit Tracker

Positive Pick New	Negative Pick Old

Use The initials of each day to track Your New & Old Habits

Water Intake	64oz. 's
Monday	
Tuesday	
Wednesday	
Thursday	
Friday	
Saturday	
Sunday	

Weekly Menu

Monday:

Tuesday:

Wednesday:

Thursday:

Friday:

Weekend:

Saturday	Sunday

Exercise/ Cardio	
Monday	
Tuesday	
Wednesday	
Thursday	
Friday	
Saturday	
Sunday	

Specify whether Cardio or Strength Training. E/C

What are some New foods you can try make a list?	Brkfast	Lunch	Dinner
Monday			
Tuesday			
Wednesday			
Thursday			
Friday			
Saturday			
Sunday			

1 hr After each meal mark how you feel as far as energy, with the New Foods from Your list !

New Habits

What are some New things that You would like to try?

1.
2.
3.

Okay Pick one & Track

M	T	W	Th	F	S	S

Put a check mark each day to track Your New Habit for the next 6 Weeks

Water Intake	64oz. 's
Week 45	
Week 46	
Week 47	
Week 48	
Week 49	

Have you been keeping up with your water intake?

Exercise/ Cardio	E	C
Week 45		
Week 46		
Week 47		
Week 48		
Week 49		

Fill in how many hours You Trained for each week

Progress Assessment

1-10 How do I feel about my progress?

How many pounds have I lost?

How many inches have I lost around my waist?

How do you look in the mirror on a scale of 1-10?

What size is your clothing now?

How has your energy been lately?

Have you been sticking to your workouts? Why?

Who have been your best Supporters?

What has been the hardest part of this journey?

What do you like most about where you are today?

December 2020

Sun	Mon	Tue	Wed	Thu	Fri	Sat
	30	1 RosaParks	2	3	4	5
6	7	8	9	10	11 Hanukkah	12
13	14	15	16	17	18 Han.Ends	19
20	21	22	23	24	25 Christmas	26 Kwanzaa
27	28	29	30	31	1 New Years	2

Monthly Overview/Notes

Put a check mark if you ate on time!	Brkfast	Lunch	Dinner
Monday			
Tuesday	✓		
Wednesday			
Thursday			
Friday			
Saturday			
Sunday			

1 hr After each meal write an emoji for how you feel as far as energy, happy for good sad for bad!

Habit Tracker

Positive Pick New	Negative Pick Old

Use The initials of each day to track Your New & Old Habits

Water Intake	64oz. 's
Monday	
Tuesday	
Wednesday	
Thursday	
Friday	
Saturday	
Sunday	

Exercise/ Cardio		
Monday		
Tuesday		
Wednesday		
Thursday		
Friday		
Saturday		
Sunday		

Specify whether Cardio or Strength Training. E/C

Weekly Menu

Monday:

Tuesday:

Wednesday:

Thursday:

Friday:

Weekend:

Saturday	Sunday

Put a check mark if you ate on time!	Brkfast		Lunch		Dinner	
Monday						
Tuesday	✓					
Wednesday						
Thursday						
Friday						
Saturday						
Sunday						

1 hr After each meal write an emoji for how you feel as far as energy, happy for good sad for bad!

Habit Tracker

Positive Pick New	Negative Pick Old

Use The initials of each day to track Your New & Old Habits

Water Intake	64oz. 's
Monday	
Tuesday	
Wednesday	
Thursday	
Friday	
Saturday	
Sunday	

Exercise/ Cardio		
Monday		
Tuesday		
Wednesday		
Thursday		
Friday		
Saturday		
Sunday		

Specify whether Cardio or Strength Training. E/C

Weekly Menu

Monday:

Tuesday:

Wednesday:

Thursday:

Friday:

Weekend:

Saturday	Sunday

Put a check mark if you ate on time!	Brkfast	Lunch	Dinner
Monday			
Tuesday			
Wednesday			
Thursday			
Friday			
Saturday			
Sunday			

1 hr After each meal write an emoji for how you feel as far as energy, happy for good sad for bad!

Habit Tracker

Positive Pick New		Negative Pick Old	
	T		
W			F

Use The initials of each day to track Your New & Old Habits

Water Intake	64oz. 's
Monday	
Tuesday	
Wednesday	
Thursday	
Friday	
Saturday	
Sunday	

Exercise/ Cardio		
Monday		
Tuesday		
Wednesday		
Thursday		
Friday		
Saturday		
Sunday		

Specify whether Cardio or Strength Training. E/C

Weekly Menu

Monday:

Tuesday:

Wednesday:

Thursday:

Friday:

Weekend:

Saturday	Sunday

Put a check mark if you ate on time!	Brkfast		Lunch		Dinner	
Monday						
Tuesday	✓					
Wednesday						
Thursday						
Friday						
Saturday						
Sunday						

1 hr After each meal write an emoji for how you feel as far as energy, happy for good sad for bad!

Habit Tracker

Positive Pick New		Negative Pick Old	
T			
W			F

Use The initials of each day to track Your New & Old Habits

Water Intake	64oz. 's
Monday	
Tuesday	
Wednesday	
Thursday	
Friday	
Saturday	
Sunday	

Exercise/ Cardio		
Monday		
Tuesday		
Wednesday		
Thursday		
Friday		
Saturday		
Sunday		

Specify whether Cardio or Strength Training. E/C

Weekly Menu

Monday:

Tuesday:

Wednesday:

Thursday:

Friday:

Weekend:

Saturday	Sunday

Put a check mark if you ate on time!	Brkfast	Lunch	Dinner
Monday			
Tuesday	✓		
Wednesday			
Thursday			
Friday			
Saturday			
Sunday			

1 hr After each meal write an emoji for how you feel as far as energy, happy for good sad for bad!

Habit Tracker

Positive Pick New	Negative Pick Old

Use The initials of each day to track Your New & Old Habits

Water Intake 64oz. 's	
Monday	
Tuesday	
Wednesday	
Thursday	
Friday	
Saturday	
Sunday	

Exercise/ Cardio		
Monday		
Tuesday		
Wednesday		
Thursday		
Friday		
Saturday		
Sunday		

Specify whether Cardio or Strength Training. E/C

Weekly Menu

Monday:

Tuesday:

Wednesday:

Thursday:

Friday:

Weekend:

Saturday	Sunday

MY

REASONS WHY I LOVE

MY

SELF

JOURNAL

Because

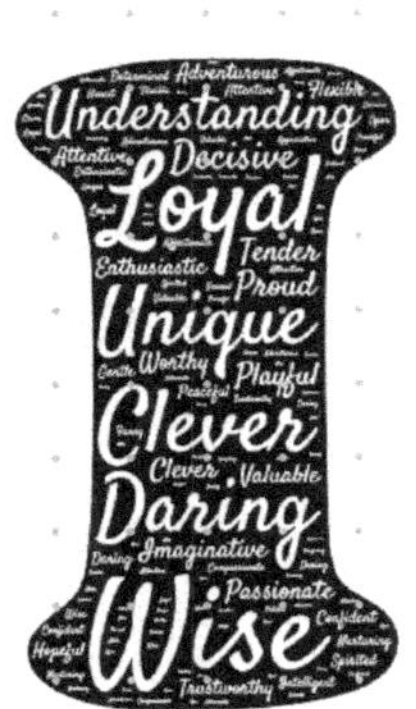

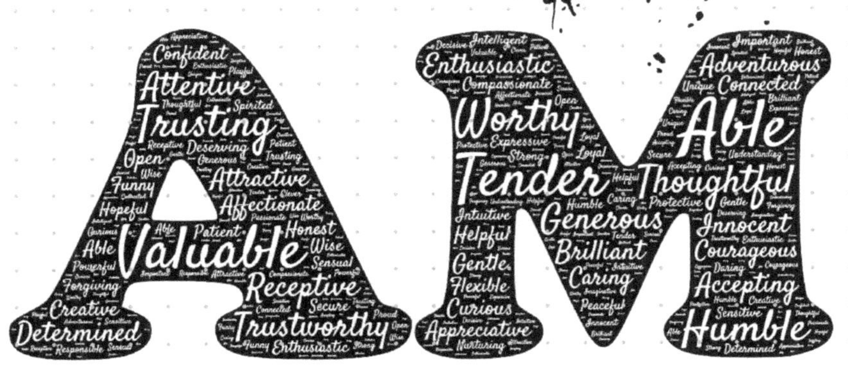

<table><tr><th>Comments/Notes</th></tr><tr><td>

</td></tr></table>

Comments/Notes

Comments/Notes

Comments/Notes

Comments/Notes

Comments/Notes

Comments/Notes

Comments/Notes

Comments/Notes

Comments/Notes

Comments/Notes

Comments/Notes

Comments/Notes

Comments/Notes

Comments/Notes

Comments/Notes

Comments/Notes

My Self Love

RECIPE BOOK

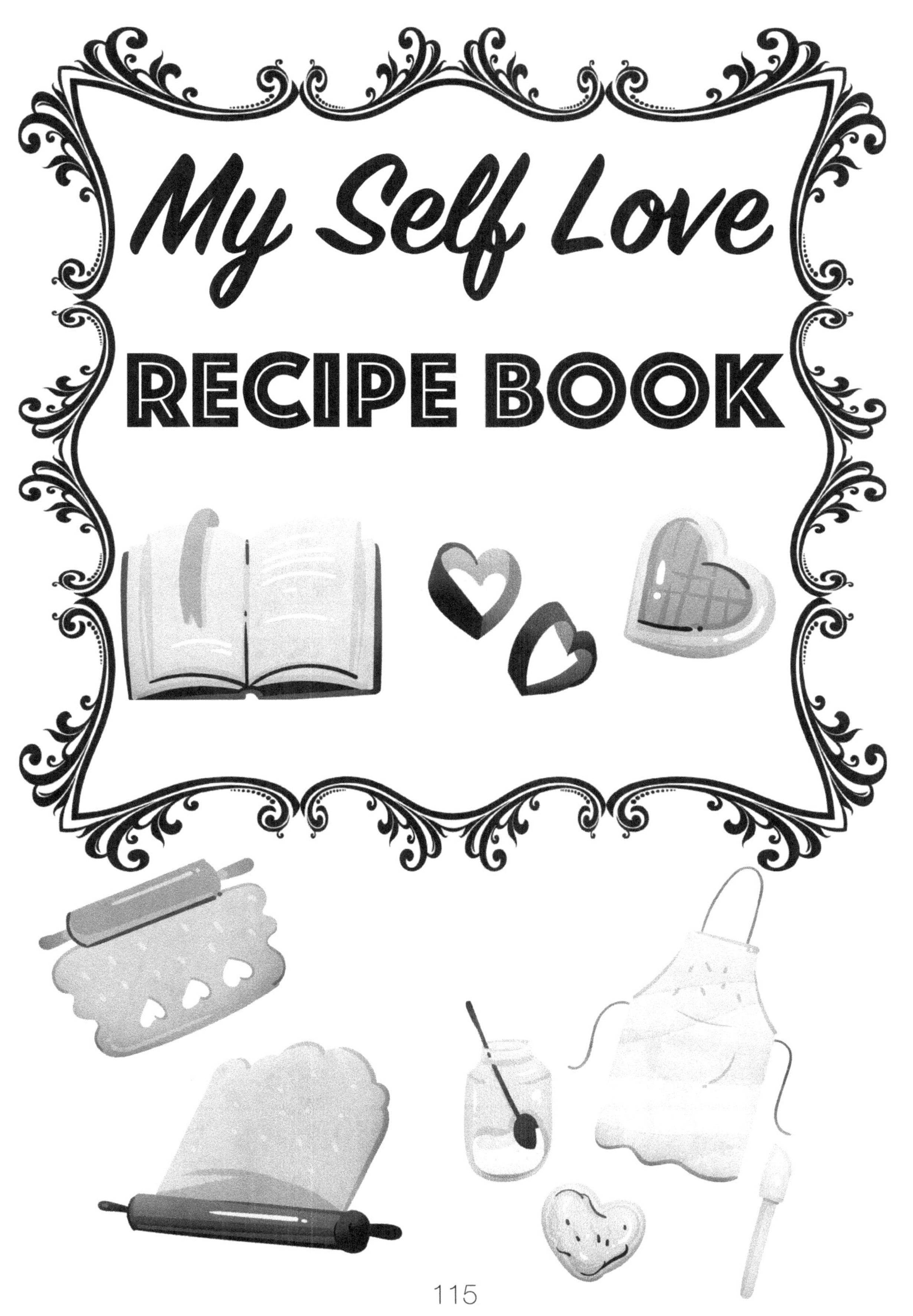

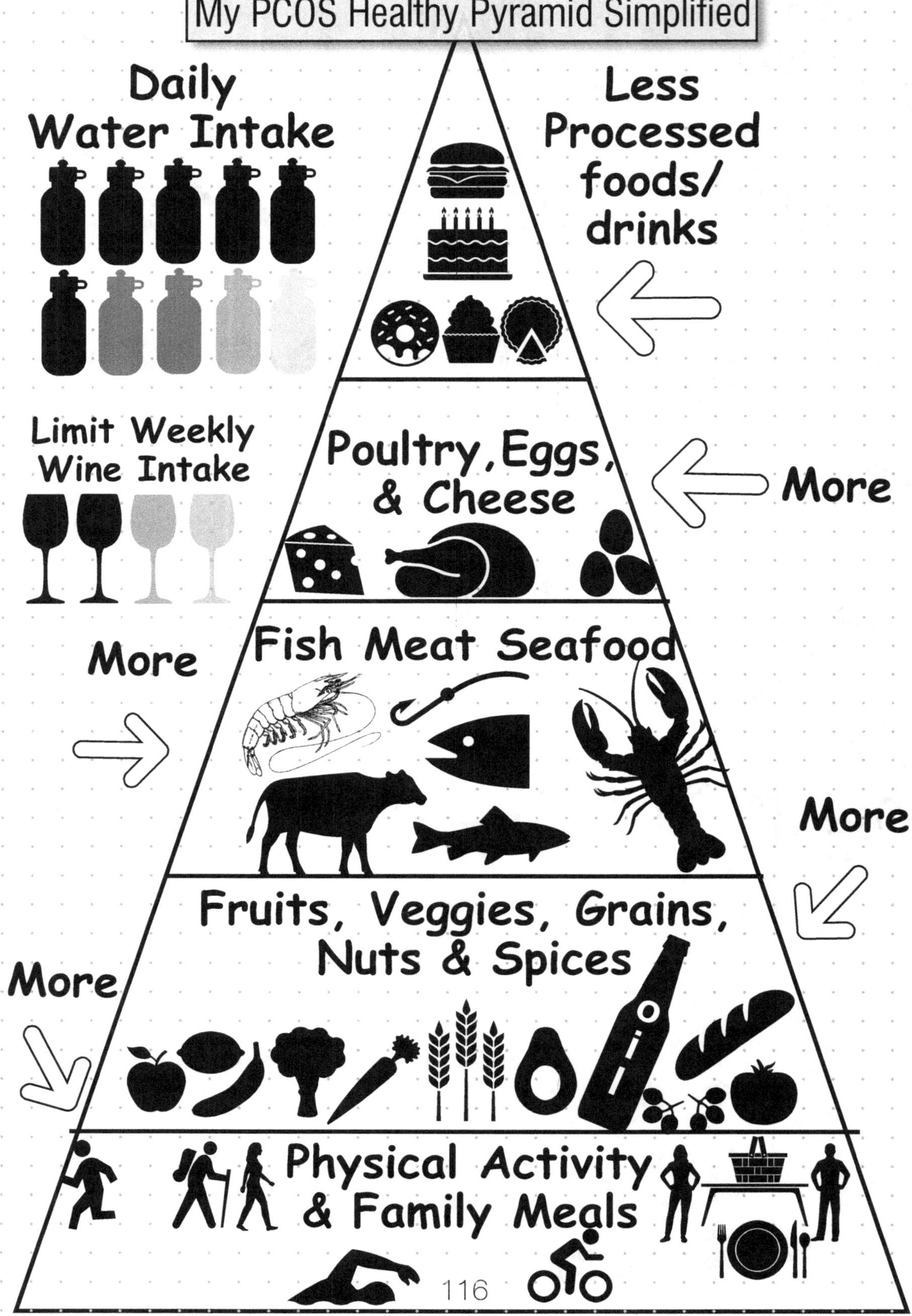

My PCOS Healthy Pyramid Simplified
Daily Water Intake
Less Processed foods/ drinks
Limit Weekly Wine Intake
Poultry, Eggs, & Cheese
More
More
Fish Meat Seafood
More
Fruits, Veggies, Grains, Nuts & Spices
More
Physical Activity & Family Meals
116

Fruit & Vegetable Starter List

6-8 per day

Apples	Broccoli	Avocado	Artichokes
Apricots	Carrots	Berries	Beets
Bananas	Cucumbers	Clementines	Cabbage
Cherries	Eggplant	Bananas	Greens
Dates	Melons	Cherries	Onions
Figs	Peaches	Pears	Pears
Grapes	Turnips	Peppers	Peas
Oranges	Yams	Tomatoes	Zucchini

Seafood & Fish Starter List

Mackerel
Bass
Cod
King Fish
Perch
Pollock
Swordfish

Herring
Mahi-mahi
Salmon
Sardines
Shark
Tuna
Trout
Snapper

Clams
Crabs
Lobster
Mussels
Oysters
Scallops
Shrimp

Herbs & Spices Starter List

Basil
Coriander
Cumin
Garlic
Mint
Rosemary
Sage
Tarragon

Allspice
Cinnamon
Nutmeg
Oregano
Parsley
Spanish Paprika

Cardamom
Cilantro
Thyme
Turmeric
Saffron
Sumac
Za'atar

Healthy Fats & Oils Starter List

3-5 x per day	3-5 x per day	1-2 x per day
Olives/Oil Nut/Butters/ Oils Fish/Oils Seed/Oils	Avocado/Oils/ Butters Coconut/MCT Oil	Yogurts Ghee Cottage Cheese

If you drink milk make it Almond (yes it's processed but you're not a calf so NO cow's milk) or something similar like rice or something.

Healthy Grains Starter List

Bulgar	Brown Rice	Rye
Buckwheat	Barley	Popcorn
Oats	Couscous	Sorghum
Farro	Millet	Maize
Polenta	Quinoa	Whole Grain
Wheat Berries	Spelt	Wild Rice

Recipe:

Serving:

Prep Time:

Cook Time:

Temperature:

Ingredients:

Methods:

Notes

Recipe:

Serving: Prep Time:

Cook Time: Temperature:

Ingredients: Methods:

Notes

Recipe: ___________________________

Serving: _________________   Prep Time: _________________

Cook Time: _______________   Temperature: _______________

Ingredients:

____

____

____

____

____

____

____

____

____

____

____

____

____

____

____

Methods:

____

____

____

____

____

____

____

____

____

____

____

____

____

____

____

Notes

____

____

Recipe:

Serving: Prep Time:

Cook Time: Temperature:

Ingredients: Methods:

Notes

Recipe: _______________________

Serving: _______________   Prep Time: _______________

Cook Time: _______________   Temperature: _______________

Ingredients:

____

Methods:

____

Notes

Recipe:

Serving: Prep Time:

Cook Time: Temperature:

Ingredients: Methods:

Notes

Recipe: ______________________________

Serving: _________________   Prep Time: _________________

Cook Time: _________________   Temperature: _________________

Ingredients:

Methods:

Notes

Recipe:

Serving:

Prep Time:

Cook Time:

Temperature:

Ingredients:

Methods:

Notes

Recipe: _______________________

Serving: _______________   Prep Time: _______________

Cook Time: _______________   Temperature: _______________

Ingredients: | Methods:

Notes

Recipe:

Serving: Prep Time:

Cook Time: Temperature:

Ingredients: Methods:

Notes

Recipe: _______________________

Serving: _______________   Prep Time: _______________

Cook Time: _______________   Temperature: _______________

Ingredients: Methods:
___________________   ___________________
___________________   ___________________
___________________   ___________________
___________________   ___________________
___________________   ___________________
___________________   ___________________
___________________   ___________________
___________________   ___________________
___________________   ___________________
___________________   ___________________
___________________   ___________________
___________________   ___________________
___________________   ___________________
___________________   ___________________
___________________   ___________________

Notes

____
____
____

Recipe:

Serving: Prep Time:

Cook Time: Temperature:

Ingredients: Methods:

Notes

Recipe:

Serving: Prep Time:

Cook Time: Temperature:

Ingredients: Methods:

Notes

Recipe: ______________________________

Serving: ______________ Prep Time: ______________

Cook Time: ______________ Temperature: ______________

Ingredients: | Methods:

Notes

Recipe:

Serving: Prep Time:

Cook Time: Temperature:

Ingredients: Methods:

Notes

Recipe: _______________________________

Serving: _______________ Prep Time: _______________

Cook Time: _______________ Temperature: _______________

Ingredients:

Methods:

Notes

Recipe:

Serving: Prep Time:

Cook Time: Temperature:

Ingredients: Methods:

Notes

Recipe:

Serving: Prep Time:

Cook Time: Temperature:

Ingredients: Methods:

Notes

Recipe: _______________________________

Serving: ___________   Prep Time: ___________

Cook Time: ___________   Temperature: ___________

Ingredients:

____
____
____
____
____
____
____
____
____
____
____
____
____
____
____
____

Methods:

____
____
____
____
____
____
____
____
____
____
____
____
____
____
____
____

Notes

____
____
____

Recipe:

Serving: Prep Time:

Cook Time: Temperature:

Ingredients: Methods:

Notes

Recipe:

Serving: Prep Time:

Cook Time: Temperature:

Ingredients: Methods:

Notes

Recipe:

Serving: Prep Time:

Cook Time: Temperature:

Ingredients: Methods:

Notes

Recipe: ______________________________

Serving: __________________   Prep Time: __________________

Cook Time: __________________   Temperature: __________________

Ingredients:

Methods:

Notes

Recipe:

Serving: Prep Time:

Cook Time: Temperature:

Ingredients: Methods:

Notes

Recipe:

Serving: Prep Time:

Cook Time: Temperature:

Ingredients: Methods:

Notes

Recipe:

Serving: Prep Time:

Cook Time: Temperature:

Ingredients: Methods:

Notes

Recipe: ______________________

Serving: ____________   Prep Time: ____________

Cook Time: ____________   Temperature: ____________

Ingredients:

____
____
____
____
____
____
____
____
____
____
____
____
____
____
____
____

Methods:

____
____
____
____
____
____
____
____
____
____
____
____
____
____
____
____

Notes

____
____

Recipe:

Serving:

Prep Time:

Cook Time:

Temperature:

Ingredients:

Methods:

Notes

Recipe:

Serving: Prep Time:

Cook Time: Temperature:

Ingredients: Methods:

Notes

Recipe:

Serving: Prep Time:

Cook Time: Temperature:

Ingredients: Methods:

Notes

www.ingramcontent.com/pod-product-compliance
Lightning Source LLC
Chambersburg PA
CBHW081722250726
48657CB00010B/3081